Nursing:

A Guide for Nurse To Flourish In Their Profession

AVALON SOULETTE BROWN, RN, BSN

Author: Avalon Soulette Brown

Published by: Avalon Soulette Brown

This book may not be reproduced in any form, retrieved, or transmitted in any form or by any means, photocopied, recordings, or otherwise without prior written permission of the publisher.

ISBN: 9798321624289

Copyright April 2024 by Avalon Soulette Brown

All rights reserved.

Printed in the United States of America

In the US write: Avalon Soulette Brown

Belleville NJ

DEDICATION

This book is dedicated to all the aspiring young women who have chosen nursing as their career path. Additionally, I extend this dedication to the nurses who have influenced and guided me throughout my journey, imparting valuable knowledge and expertise in various specialty areas. I am immensely grateful for the skills and growth I have acquired through their mentorship. Their willingness to share their wisdom has shaped me into the nurse I am today. To those who recognized my potential and supported my advancement to leadership roles, whether as a charge person, manager, or leader among peers, I express my heartfelt gratitude. This dedication is a tribute to each of you.

TABLE OF CONTENTS

INTRODUCTION

Chapter I..1

KEY STEPS TO PREPARE FOR A CAREER IN NURSING

Chapter II..8

HAVING GOOD MENTORSHIP IN NURSING

Chapter III..16

HOW TO PRIORITIZE YOUR WORKLOAD IN NURSING

Chapter IV..23

HOW TO BE AN EFFECTIVE TEAM MEMBER

Chapter V...29

SHOWING EMPATHY & COMPASSION AS A NURSE

Chapter VI..34

HOW TO HAVE FLEXIBILITY AS A NURSING

Chapter VII 40

HOW CONTINUING EDUCATION HELP NURSES?

Chapter VIII..48

ETHICAL AND LEGAL CONSIDERATIONS IN NURSING

Chapter IX.. 52

NAVIGATING THE PATH OF NURSING ENTREPRENEURSHIP

Chapter X...55

THE BUSINESS THAT ALMOST WAS

ACKNOWLEDGMENT

First, I want to acknowledge God who granted me the strength courage to complete 42 years of nursing. It was his guidance that watched over me. through every challenge I faced and overcame. Thank you.

Next, I want to express my gratitude to all the nurses who helped shape me. into the nurse I am today. They dedicated their time and patience to an impart. their knowledge, enabling me to thrive in my career. I also want to acknowledge my supervisors for recognizing and elevating my potential. throughout my career.

Lastly, I extend my thanks to my children, grandchildren, and great. Grandchildren. for their unwavering support. Your encouragement means everything to me. Thank you, everyone for being part of my journey

INTRODUCTION

In the dynamic and demanding field of healthcare, nurses play a crucial role in ensuring the well-being of patients and contributing to the overall effectiveness of medical teams. Flourishing as a nurse involves a combination of professional development, compassionate care, and maintaining a healthy work-life balance. Firstly, continuous education is key to staying abreast of the latest medical advancements and enhancing clinical skills. Pursuing additional certifications, attending workshops, and participating in ongoing training programs not only broadens a nurse's knowledge base but also opens opportunities for career growth.

Secondly, the heart of nursing lies in compassionate patient care. Building strong interpersonal relationships, practicing empathy, and maintaining effective communication with both patients and their families foster a supportive and healing environment. A flourishing nurse understands the importance of holistic care, addressing not only the physical but also the emotional and psychological needs of patients. This compassionate approach not only positively impacts patient outcomes but also contributes to a more fulfilling and meaningful nursing career.

Lastly, achieving balance between professional responsibilities and personal well-being is essential for sustained success in nursing. Nurses often face high-stress situations, long hours, and emotionally challenging experiences. Prioritizing self-care, setting realistic boundaries, and seeking support from colleagues and mentors contribute to a resilient and flourishing nursing career. By embracing these principles of continuous learning, compassionate care, and self-care, nurses can navigate the complexities of their profession and find fulfillment in their essential role within the healthcare system.

CHAPTER I

HOW TO PREPARE FOR A CAREER IN NURSING?

INTRODUCTION

Before deciding to pursue a career in nursing, it is important to thoroughly investigate if this is truly the path you want to take. You should consider several factors before enrolling in school, such as whether nursing aligns with your passion, the time commitment required for nursing education, and the content of the nursing curriculum.

.

What Is the Significance of Researching The P Nursing Profession?

Thorough research into the nursing profession is a critical and foundational step for individuals considering a career in this field. This involves a comprehensive exploration of relevant literature, including articles and books, to gain an in-depth understanding of the profession's intricacies. Documentation of findings is essential to facilitate an informed decision-making process. Additionally, prospective nurses should carefully evaluate various educational institutions, scrutinizing school curriculums and ensuring accreditation status. Acquiring precise knowledge about the duration of the educational journey, types of nursing degrees, and specific prerequisites is imperative. Deliberate planning regarding the preferred degree, duration of the program, required classes, and prerequisites is essential to avoid unnecessary financial and temporal investments. Thorough research serves as a prudent approach to ensure that individuals enter the nursing profession with a comprehensive understanding, minimizing the risk of making uninformed decisions that may lead to dissatisfaction or a mismatch between personal aspirations and the realities of the profession.

As a young child, I developed a fondness for watching TV, particularly hospital shows from years ago. It was during this time that I made the decision to pursue a career in nursing. I was captivated by the sight of nurses in their white caps, white shoes, and white uniforms, which left a deep impression on me. This moment ignited a passion within me to care for others, a desire that persisted throughout my years in grade and high school. Upon reaching high school, I sought guidance from counselors and applied to several nursing programs. After graduating, I was accepted into a college located in a neighboring town. This marked the beginning of my journey to achieve my goals in nursing.

.

What Is The Importance of Discussing The Nursing Profession With Other Nurses?

If you possess a genuine interest in nursing, it would be advisable to engage in conversations with seasoned nurses who have accumulated a year or more of experience in the field. Seek their insights on various aspects such as their overall perspective on working as a nurse, job satisfaction, and their sentiments towards their profession. Inquiring about their level of contentment and passion for their work can provide valuable insights. Evaluating whether pursuing a career in nursing is a worthwhile endeavor can be better assessed through such discussions. Establishing communication with fellow nurses is pivotal, as they can offer diverse perspectives, especially across different specialties within the nursing profession. This will allow you to make informed decisions and potentially identify a specific field within nursing that aligns with your preferences.

During my first year at college, a friend of mine helped me secure a job in a hospital working in dietary services. This opportunity allowed me to observe nurses up close and interact with them while distributing patient trays. I noticed how tirelessly they worked, constantly moving up and down the halls. Although they had limited time for conversation, I often stopped to chat with the nurse's aides. They shared stories about their experiences working on the units, but instead of deterring me, it strengthened my resolve to pursue nursing as my career goal. Engaging in conversations with experienced professionals in various nursing specialties is essential for making informed decisions about one's career path.

Why Is It Important To Know Your Level of Resilience To Stressful Situations?

"Nursing is widely recognized for its demanding and potentially stressful nature. Recognizing and acknowledging your own level of resilience is a key for preparing for the daily rigors of nursing. This self-awareness equips nurses to effectively handle distressing situations, ensuring the completion of tasks and fulfilling their duties with competence and professionalism." In the face of adversity, resilience becomes a cornerstone, ensuring that individuals can effectively manage the difficulties that may arise. It is imperative for nurses to possess the strength and determination not to succumb to the urge to quit when confronted with challenging situations.

"There have been numerous instances when I faced challenges, including tight schedules and demanding assignments that significantly increased my workload. Despite having to work through these situations, I persevered and continued to work diligently. For example, there were occasions where I had a high patient load and insufficient support on the floor, with just two aides available. The challenge emerged in having to distribute these two aides among two or three nurses, resulting in a slowdown in productivity. However, having the strength to persist in such situations is where resilience plays a crucial role. You do not want to be that person who gives up when every unpleasant situation gets to be overwhelming.

Not every day in nursing is smooth; there are days filled with challenges. It's essential to acknowledge that your days won't always be easy, but it's about making the best of the circumstances. There are times when workload and staffing constraints will impede progress, making it challenging to complete tasks. The key is to maintain resilience and press on. Giving up is not an option in the face of a stressful day, as nursing inherently involves stress. It's crucial to assess your ability to cope with such situations and recognize that resilience is an integral aspect of successfully navigating the demanding nature of the profession."

Why Is It Important To Know Your Long-term Goals Professionally and Personally?

When deciding to enter the nursing field, it is crucial to define your goals and expectations. Consider where you see yourself in the next five years. Establishing specific goals for your nursing career can significantly contribute to your success in a particular specialty. Whether your aim is to enter management, work in the ICU, focus on trauma, work in the emergency room, or outpatient care, having clear goals provides a direction for your post-education journey. By setting these goals, you can actively work towards these certifications, educational classes, or webinars. Reflecting on my own experience, I entered nursing without specific goals, leading to an eighteen-year career in areas such as Med Surg, then twenty years in dialysis, and three-and-a-half-year infection control. If you're entering nursing with a preference for a particular specialty, setting goals allows you to focus your efforts and pursue the career path that aligns with your aspirations.

As I embarked on my nursing career, my personal goals are intricately tied to both my professional aspirations and the responsibilities in my personal life, particularly as a parent. I recognize the importance of setting realistic and achievable goals that align with the demands of nursing practice while considering the needs of my family. One of my primary objectives was to have a balance between work and family life, ensuring the hours and days I needed. By the time I started working as a nurse I was already a parent and because I was a parent it was ideal for me to start working on the night shift. When my children became old enough to be able to walk to school together, I transferred to the day shift. Additionally, I excelled in my nursing role by continuously enhancing my skills and staying updated on advancements in healthcare, all while being mindful of how my professional pursuits can positively impact my family. By setting these goals, I was able to create a harmonious integration of my nursing career and personal life.

During my time in the nursing program, I didn't have a specific specialty area that I was determined to pursue. I initially began in Med-Surg because there was an opening for a position there. Over the course of 18 years in that field, I developed an interest in dialysis, eventually spending 20 years working in that area before transitioning into infection control. These specialty areas weren't my initial goals when I started as a new nurse; they simply evolved over time as opportunities arose.

What Should You Know About Licensing, Certificates, and Degrees in Nursing?

Gain a comprehensive understanding of the procedural steps and examinations essential for obtaining a nursing license. Stay updated on any changes or revisions in licensing procedures to ensure strict adherence to regulatory standards. It is particularly crucial to be well-versed in the process of obtaining a license, especially if there are potential plans for relocating to another state, or work as a travel nurse in the future. Investigate the unique licensure requirements of each state, explore the possibility of acquiring a dual license to practice in two states without the need for additional exams, and consider reciprocity options. It is imperative to identify which states accept multi-state licensure to facilitate a smooth transition. Following successful completion of the license exam, familiarize yourself with the policies governing your license. Drawing from personal experience,

I initially started as a Licensed Practical Nurse (LPN) in the eighties, a period during which LPNs faced certain restrictions. Consequently, I diligently reviewed the guidelines for LPNs to ensure strict adherence to my scope of practice. Recognize that the LPN license operates under the umbrella of the Registered Nurse (RN) license, providing opportunities for roles such as a charge nurse. However, it is essential to understand and adhere to all requirements and guidelines stipulated by the Board of Nursing under your specific licensure category.

It's important to be aware of the various levels of nursing degrees available, including the associate degree, bachelor's degree, master's degree, and doctorate. If you opt for an associate degree, the program typically spans two years, while a bachelor's degree requires a four-year commitment. One notable distinction among these degrees is the potential impact on your pay rate, your eligibility for leadership roles, and the specific nursing positions you may pursue. Your choice of nursing degree can significantly influence your career trajectory and opportunities within the field.

While having the highest degree in nursing can certainly be advantageous, what I've learned over the years is that timing and circumstances also play a significant role. Throughout my practice, there was always the belief that a bachelor's degree was necessary to become a charge nurse or clinical manager. However, I achieved the role of clinical manager with an associate degree. This illustrates that the requirements can vary depending on the facility, the organization, or the individuals in leadership positions. Regardless of your nursing degree level, you can still make valuable contributions to improving the quality of care.

CHAPTER II

HAVING GOOD MENTORSHIP IN NURSING

INTRODUCTION

Mentorship plays a pivotal role in the nursing profession, providing a vital support system for both new and experienced nurses. In the demanding field of healthcare, mentorship fosters professional development, knowledge transfer, and skill enhancement. For new nurses, mentors serve as invaluable guides, offering insights into the intricacies of patient care, ethical considerations, and the complex healthcare environment. Mentorship enhances the overall quality of patient care by promoting a culture of continuous learning and fostering a sense of community within the nursing workforce. In a rapidly evolving healthcare landscape, the importance of mentorship cannot be overstated, as it not only contributes to the growth of individual nurses but also strengthens the fabric of the nursing profession.

What Steps Ensure a Successful Transition from Student Nurse to Professional Nurse?

Upon obtaining your nursing license and embarking on your professional journey, you will undergo a crucial mentoring period lasting approximately 6 to 8 weeks. During this time, your assigned preceptor will work closely with you on a day-to-day basis, systematically guiding you through the intricacies of the unit's routine. This mentoring process involves a comprehensive overview of policies and procedures, introductions to team members, and gradual acclimatization to the unit's operational dynamics.

Reflecting on my own entry into nursing, I encountered a challenge on my initial unit where the head nurse perceived me to have an attitude issue. However, my reserved demeanor stemmed from a sincere focus on learning the unit's routine. Consequently, I transitioned to another unit where the head nurse served as my mentor. She fostered a supportive environment, avoiding any form of reprimand, and facilitated my understanding of the floor's intricacies.

Transitioning from being a student to assuming the role of a nurse stirred up a sense of nervousness within me. While in school, there's a certain comfort in being guided by a teacher and having clear expectations set. However, as a nurse on the unit, without that constant guidance, my confidence initially wavered. Now, I find myself entrusted with a license that I must diligently protect, a responsibility that reinforces my commitment to my profession.

In a subsequent shift to the night schedule, I found mentorship from two Filipino nurses who graciously took me under their wing. They imparted invaluable knowledge encompassing floor processes, policies, patient care, treatments, and medication administration. One of these nurses, formerly a nursing educator in her home country, exhibited remarkable patience and dedication in sharing her extensive expertise. I can say they help make me the nurse I am today.

Why Is It Important to Have A Positive Learning Environment?

This experience underscores the significance of having a preceptor who invests time, patience, and a comfortable learning environment. It is imperative to identify a mentor who not only imparts knowledge but also instills confidence, ensuring a seamless transition into the nursing profession. In the role of a preceptor, it is crucial to establish a positive training environment characterized by patience, encouragement, and the willingness to address numerous inquiries. Devoting extra attention to areas of weakness and facilitating an open dialogue are essential aspects of effective training. As a trainee, it is encouraged to actively seek guidance, and the preceptor's approachability plays a pivotal role in fostering an environment where questions can be freely posed.

Drawing from my personal experience as a trained preceptor, I prioritized creating an inclusive atmosphere with an open-door policy, allowing new nurses to feel at ease while learning various tasks. Balancing a friendly demeanor with a professional approach, a preceptor should maintain a welcoming and caring attitude. Addressing any concerns promptly by communicating with the appropriate authority is advised to ensure a comfortable and conducive learning environment. A preceptor's guidance should encompass a structured orientation list, providing a clear roadmap for the trainee's development on a week-by-week and day-by-day basis. This structured approach enables trainees to anticipate expectations and take proactive steps in their learning journey. Establishing and maintaining a positive learning environment is paramount, as it significantly contributes to the effectiveness of the training process and the trainee's ability to grasp essential tasks.

When I chose to transition into a different nursing specialty, I opted to become a dialysis nurse due to my longstanding interest in the field. This interest stemmed from my experiences on our med-surge unit, where we frequently referred patients to dialysis early in the morning.

Upon noticing an advertisement seeking nurses for outpatient clients, I decided to apply despite lacking prior experience, as the ad indicated they would provide training. Following a four-week training period, I commenced working on the floor. The charge nurse demonstrated exceptional patience with me, recognizing my initial struggles. She reassured me that it was okay to take time to learn and encouraged me to persist, assuring me that I would eventually grasp the concepts.

It took me six months to feel confident working independently without supervision, and I credit this achievement to the supportive and nurturing environment created by that charge nurse.

Why Is It Important to Promote Independence During Mentorship?

When being mentored, it is crucial that your independence is fostered when being guided as a new nurse through training. You have already completed your educational training, obtained your license, and received their diploma. Therefore, it is essential to provide you with the space to highlight their knowledge. Your mentor should offer encouragement while you carry out your assigned tasks. Rather than actively managing every aspect, your mentor should step back and assess your capabilities. Provide a list of expected tasks and observe which ones you can execute independently. While you may require guidance and have questions, it's important for the mentor to refrain from excessive micromanagement. Offer initial demonstrations, and then allow you the autonomy to perform tasks on your own. Observe your execution, noting correct actions and identifying any missed steps. Granting you this level of independence during training not only instills a sense of fulfillment but also boosts your confidence and motivates you to take on more responsibilities. Avoiding excessive micromanagement is crucial, as it allows the mentor to discern your strengths and weaknesses, helping you prioritize areas that require additional focus during your training.

In my role as a trained preceptor, I prefer using a structured approach during orientation. This involves informing them about the duration of the orientation help sessions, discussing the integration plan weekly, outlining the tasks and learning objectives for each week, and demonstrating the tasks initially before stepping back to assess their understanding. I encourage questions and aim to instill confidence in their abilities, leveraging their clinical experience from nursing studies to demonstrate how theoretical knowledge translates into practice.

However, it's crucial for every nurse to recognize the importance of following the orientation process, adhering to facility policies and procedures, and understanding the specific protocols of their workplace. While I maintain a hands-off approach, giving them space to work independently, I remain observant to evaluate their retention of knowledge from school and their adherence to the orientation program's timelines. This strategic distance allows them to demonstrate their capabilities while ensuring they receive necessary guidance and support.

This approach aims to instill a sense of autonomy in their tasks, all the while keenly watching for potential errors or mistakes. The intention is not to micromanage, as this can induce nervousness in the trainee, leading to a lack of confidence and an increased likelihood of mistakes. Instead, the goal is to strike a balance where the trainee feels empowered and confident in executing the assigned tasks.

Why Encourage Critical Think During Your Mentorship?

Encouraging critical thinking skills is paramount in nursing as it fosters a dynamic and proactive approach to patient care. As a nurse, you must go beyond rote memorization and routine procedures to navigate the complex and ever-evolving healthcare landscape. One effective strategy to stimulate critical thinking is for your mentor to present you with a challenging case scenario, urging you to analyze and synthesize information from various sources. This not only enhances your problem-solving abilities but also sharpens your clinical judgment. Encouraging open-ended discussions during team meetings or training sessions allows you to express your perspectives and engage in collaborative thinking, promoting a culture where diverse viewpoints contribute to well-rounded decision-making.

When being trained as a new nurse, it becomes crucial to expose you to diverse situations and challenges. For instance, when addressing patient scenarios, it is beneficial to present you with specific problems related to the patient's condition. By doing so, you can evaluate your problem-solving approach and inquire about the steps they would take in resolving these issues. Additionally, tailoring the questions to the specific nursing specialty being covered in the training is essential, given the diverse areas within the field of nursing. Engaging the trainee in problem-solving exercises allows you to assess your capabilities and ask for guidance as needed. This presents an opportunity for further training, where you can get assistance in understanding any incorrect answers, addressing questions, and elucidating the correct solutions. As a mentor, their role should involve facilitating this learning process and providing a platform for you to ask questions, clarify misconceptions, and enhance your problem-solving skills within your designated nursing specialty.

When I precept or mentor a new nurse during orientation, I find it crucial to engage you in critical thinking. Instead of simply demonstrating tasks, I prompt you to consider the why behind your actions, the desired outcomes, and the reasons for your procedures. I create scenarios to encourage you to think about your decision-making processes and objectives. If you encounter a question and you don't know the answer to, I suggest taking notes or using a tablet to look up the information later.

Sometimes, we pause to find the answer together during the training session, while other times, I ask you to research and provide the answer during the next session. This approach fosters a deeper understanding of the tasks and encourages independent problem-solving skills, ensuring you can apply their knowledge effectively in various situations.

What specific skills or knowledge have I gained from my mentorship experience?

During orientation, pausing to evaluate what you have learned or retained from your mentorship is beneficial. This assessment enables you to identify your strengths and weaknesses, pinpoint areas needing improvement, and seek additional training if necessary. Additionally, providing feedback to your mentor helps them continue supporting you in reaching your goals.

In every nursing specialty I worked in, I made sure to express gratitude to my mentor for all the valuable lessons I learned. Transitioning from inpatient to outpatient nursing, I brought with me eighteen years of nursing experience. However, in outpatient nursing, I realized the need to adapt my entire thought process, especially during dialysis. For instance, in inpatient nursing, we are cautious when a patient has a central line to avoid rapid fluid infusion initially. In contrast, I learned in dialysis that when a patient's blood pressure drops, it's necessary to infuse fluids rapidly. I am grateful to my mentor for enlightening me about the underlying concept behind this difference in fluid management.

How Do You Ensure Accountability as A Team Member?

Take ownership of your responsibilities and commitments within the team. Deliver high-quality work, meet deadlines, and fulfill your role to the best of your abilities. Hold yourself accountable for your actions and decisions and be proactive in addressing any issues or obstacles that may arise. As a team member it is important that you are accountable for your action. Whether the outcome is good or bad. Be accountable for your workload. When given assignments project try to complete them on time.

It is beneficial to outline your needs for a project and determine the timeline for completion upon receiving an appointment. I have always treated my assignments like a race against time, striving to finish them promptly and diligently. Accountability is essential in ensuring timely completion, both individually and as a team member. Collaborating with others on assignments or projects requires fulfilling your responsibilities promptly, especially when different team members handle various sections. In nursing school, I experienced successful online project collaboration by dividing tasks, appointing a leader, and completing our respective parts. This approach facilitated easy assembly of the final project from everyone's contributions.

Nurses are accountable for their attendance, callouts, and punctuality at work, along with maintaining accountability for their conduct as team members, thereby upholding nursing ethics.

CHAPTER III

HOW TO PRIORITIZE YOUR WORKLOAD IN NURSING

INTRODUCTION

In the dynamic and demanding field of nursing, effective prioritization is a critical skill that can significantly impact patient care and overall job satisfaction. Nurses are often faced with a multitude of tasks, from administering medications to coordinating patient care plans, and the ability to prioritize effectively is essential for maintaining both individual and team efficiency. This guide aims to provide valuable insights and practical strategies on how to navigate the complexities of a nursing workload, ensuring that important tasks are addressed promptly and efficiently. By honing the skill of prioritization, nurses can enhance patient outcomes, reduce stress, and contribute to a more organized and fulfilling work environment. Join us as we delve into the art of prioritizing in nursing, equipping you with the tools and mindset needed to navigate the challenges of your daily responsibilities with confidence and competence.

How To Collaborate with The Health Care Team On Your Unit?

After completing the 6 to 8 weeks of orientation, you are now transitioning to working independently. It is crucial at this stage to foster collaboration with your healthcare team. While your preceptor may be occupied, building a rapport with other team members on the unit is essential. This enables you to seek assistance, ask questions, and receive support with tasks during shift changes and patient assignments.

When receiving reports on your patients during these transitions, meticulous notetaking is imperative. Ensure you comprehend the information shared by your colleagues about the previous shift. If there is any uncertainty, do not hesitate to ask questions, as once the shift concludes, reaching out to the person may not be feasible until the next day or subsequent shift. Therefore, establishing connections with the entire care team on the floor is invaluable. Each team member contributes a unique piece to the puzzle, offering insights and advice that can significantly enhance the smoothness of your work. Collaboration within the team leads to a more effective and cohesive work environment.

When collaborating with other team members, it's important to recognize that each person has their own unique style of working and routines. Avoid dismissing their training methods by comparing them to your mentor's approach. Instead, view it as an opportunity to learn and potentially adopt different styles in the future. When working with your mentor, focus on practicing the tasks as they have instructed you. Avoid mixing the training styles of other team members during your orientation, as your mentor will evaluate you based on their teachings. This approach will also prevent confusion and ensure a clear understanding of expectations.

I recall working on a unit that welcomed new graduate nurses, and I found myself as the only seasoned nurse on that shift. Despite this, we established a strong rapport, ensuring that each team member was well-informed about the status of every patient. This way, when we took breaks, we could effectively report off, and in the presence of a doctor, we could promptly provide updates on each patient. This underscores the significance of collaborating with other team members, as it ensures there is always someone available to share information about your patient when the need arises for you to step away.

What Is The Significance of Addressing Patients' Needs and Preferences?

Addressing patients' needs and preferences is a crucial aspect of providing quality healthcare. As you begin your shift, it becomes essential to prioritize the diverse needs and preferences of each patient under your care. Every patient presents unique requirements, and it is your responsibility to discern which needs and preferences should take precedence. During the shift handover, the previous nurse will provide insights into the current condition of the patients, offering a starting point for your assessment.

Upon reviewing your assignment, consider factors such as the patient's medical needs, prescribed medications, scheduled treatments, and any upcoming diagnostic tests or X-rays. Prioritizing your day based on these factors ensures that you address the most critical needs first. Understanding where each patient needs to go and what tasks are associated with each room is equally important. In a typical assignment with 6 to 8 patients, evaluating and prioritizing the needs of everyone helps in determining the order of patient visits, optimizing efficiency, and ensuring that you allocate sufficient time to those who require more attention.

Upon receiving the shift change report from the previous nurse, I carefully considered every detail provided about the patient. Prior to addressing any other tasks, I promptly completed my rounds and conducted a comprehensive assessment for peace of mind. I engaged with each patient on my assignment to ascertain their needs and determine any scheduled tests or procedures. This approach provided me with a clear understanding of priorities and whom I needed to attend to first.

What Are Steps for Prioritizing Time Sensitive Tasks

When given a nursing assignment, it is crucial to prioritize tasks by first assessing what needs immediate attention. Determine which tests and treatments are imperative and must be conducted promptly, distinguishing them from those that can be scheduled later in the day. Prioritizing different treatments is essential, never forgetting the critical medications that must be administered. Additionally, if there is any urgent blood work, it is crucial to identify and prioritize those cases. Checking which patients require immediate treatments and understanding the timing of each treatment is vital. By prioritizing time-sensitive tasks such as medication administration, hanging medications, and scheduling tests, you can efficiently organize your entire day and workload around these priorities.:

Time-sensitive tasks in nursing are critical activities that must be performed promptly to ensure the well-being of patients. Here are examples of such tasks:

1. Medication Administration: To maintain therapeutic levels in the patient's system.

2. Vital Sign Monitoring: Regular monitoring of vital signs, heart rate, blood pressure, and resp.

3. Emergency Response: Responding quickly to emergency situations.

4. Blood Transfusions: Initiating and monitoring blood transfusions.

5 Scheduled Procedures: Preparing patients for scheduled procedures, surgeries, or diagnostic tests at the designated times.

6. Wound Care: Changing dressings and performing wound care.

7. Insulin Administration: Administering insulin injections at specific.

8. Antibiotic Administration: Ensuring timely administration of antibiotics to treat infections.

9. Intravenous (IV) Fluid Management: Monitoring and adjusting intravenous fluid rates .

10. Diagnostic Tests: Coordinating and facilitating time-sensitive diagnostic tests, such as CT scans, MRIs, or laboratory tests, to assist in diagnosis and treatment planning.

11. Postoperative Care: Monitoring and managing patients in the postoperative period.

12. Seizure Management: Administering antiepileptic medications promptly during seizures.

Timely execution of these tasks is crucial for providing effective patient care and ensuring positive health outcomes. Hopefully, you are fortunate enough to secure a routine, where you know precisely what tasks await you from the moment you arrive until you go home. It is imperative to maintain organization. Personally, I find immense value in such a structure, as it enables me to manage my time efficiently. By adhering to a clear schedule, I can ensure that all my responsibilities are completed without feeling overwhelmed. Being organized is a key attribute in nursing, as it allows for the prioritization of tasks and the ability to plan. This approach not only facilitates effective time management but also contributes to providing optimal patient care and ensuring positive health outcomes.

How Delegating Appropriately Can Help Prioritize Your Workload?

When you begin your shift, the initial step is to assess your tasks. Prioritize what needs to be done, understanding that collaboration is key. New nurses often find it helpful to enlist the support of nursing assistants. Identify the tasks within their scope and delegate, accordingly, freeing yourself to focus on higher-level responsibilities. Working in tandem fosters efficiency; there's no need to shoulder everything alone. Nursing assistants excel at handling routine tasks like patient care and logistics, allowing nurses to concentrate on more complex duties. Recognize the importance of teamwork; it's not about doing it all yourself, but rather leveraging each team member's skills effectively. Remember, delegation isn't about diminishing others but optimizing resources for better patient outcomes. Ensure clear communication and expectations, understanding that accountability rests with the nurse, even when tasks are delegated.

By establishing this collaborative approach early on, you can effectively manage your workload and provide quality care throughout your shift. When some nurses hesitate to approach their nursing assistants due to fear of pushback, it's crucial to take swift action. Remember, the **assistants** work under your license, making you responsible for patient outcomes. If they resist cooperation, it's necessary to escalate the issue by reporting them to the manager, who can address the situation appropriately.

When I started as a new nurse on the unit, I worked alongside aides who had been there for twenty years or more. They often pushed back or disappeared from the units. As I became familiar with their routines, I learned to prioritize tasks, completing what I could and saving non-urgent tasks for the aides. In my role as a mentor, I trained new nurses to be observant and encouraged them to speak up when necessary. However, I observed that the aides were delegating their tasks to the new nurses, leading to backlogs in documentation and other responsibilities.

Why Is Managing Self-Care Important?

Managing self-care is pivotal when you're responsible for both your well-being and that of your patients. While not everyone may prioritize breakfast, it served as a vital energy boost for me before commencing work. This sustenance was essential in navigating the morning's demands, from administering treatments and medications to liaising with colleagues and physicians. Neglecting self-care can lead to burnout, exacerbated by the relentless pace of hospital duties, extended shifts, and heavy patient caseloads. Regular check-ups with a primary care physician are imperative for maintaining one's health.

Adopting healthy eating habits, ensuring sufficient rest, and incorporating physical activity into daily routines can mitigate stress and enhance mood and vitality. Seeking support from peers, friends, or professional counselors is crucial when confronting workplace challenges that spill into personal life, safeguarding against burnout and depression. Allocating time outside of work for hobbies like reading or playing musical instruments fosters relaxation and rejuvenation. Amidst the demands of patient care, it's essential to carve out moments for brief respites, such as taking lunch breaks, which not only nourish the body but also prevent burnout. Establishing efficient systems allows for completing tasks promptly without undue strain, ensuring a timely departure from work and safeguarding one's well-being.

Therefore, prioritizing self-care is fundamental to sustaining effectiveness and preventing exhaustion in the demanding healthcare environment. Ensuring I took my lunch break was a consistent practice of mine. This emphasizes the value of teamwork, as it allows for tasks to be delegated among team members. By effectively communicating the status of assignments to colleagues, any arising issues can be addressed even when one is temporarily off the unit.

CHAPTER IV

HOW TO BE AN EFFECTIVE TEAM MEMBER

INTRODUCTION

In today's dynamic and interconnected world, success often hinges on our ability to collaborate effectively within teams. Whether in the workplace, academia, or community initiatives, the power of teamwork cannot be overstated. Yet, being an effective team member is not merely about showing up and fulfilling assigned tasks; it's about actively contributing, communicating, and synergizing with fellow members to achieve collective goals.

This chapter delves into the intricacies of what it takes to be an exemplary team member. From fostering open communication to nurturing a collaborative spirit, each facet plays a pivotal role in the overall success of the team. While individual skills and talents are valuable, it's the cohesive effort of every team member that propels projects forward and facilitates innovation.

Why Is Communication Important As A Team Member?

Effective communication within a team is crucial for fostering a productive workflow and minimizing conflicts. It involves articulating ideas clearly and precisely, while also being receptive to others' perspectives without judgment. Responding positively to feedback and maintaining an appropriate tone are essential components of successful communication. If communication presents a challenge, seeking out communication services, seminars, or webinars can be beneficial. Additionally, ensuring that written communication is clear and legible for all team members is essential. Communication should be tailored to be understandable by all members of the multidisciplinary team, facilitating cohesion and efficient delegation of tasks. Unification through clear and effective communication is key to successful teamwork, as it enables transparency and shared understanding of goals, tasks, and responsibilities. As a team leader or manager, it is crucial to communicate with your team in a friendly tone. Communication delivered in an intimidating manner can diminish your team members' enthusiasm for completing their assignments. Precise and clear written communication is also important. The reader must be clear with the message or written report you are conveying.

When I was a charge nurse, my aim was to communicate with the team in a manner that would motivate them to willingly work overtime or take on extra assignments. The way you communicate can significantly affect whether the job is enjoyable or if the staff feels miserable. In cases of disagreements with your teammates, shouting and screaming at each other should never occur. Conflict resolution is more effective when each party remains calm and speaks in an acceptable tone. Unwanted communication may result in written disciplinary actions.

Why Is It Important To Respect Everyone In The Team?

Respecting every member of the multidisciplinary team is paramount. Within such a diverse cultural context, it's crucial to acknowledge and honor various cultural norms, including language, cuisine, and communication styles. Each team member brings a unique blend of skills, experiences, and perspectives to the table, emphasizing the importance of being an attentive listener when they express their ideas or present projects. Maintaining respectful communication among team members is essential; refrain from raising voices or engaging in unprofessional behavior during conflicts. Disrespect towards team members can negatively impact team cohesion and retention, potentially leading to the departure of valuable members. When faced with disrespectful behavior, it's essential to address it promptly, whether by discussing it with the individual directly or bringing it to the attention of the appropriate authority for resolution. By fostering a culture of mutual respect, teams can thrive and collaborate effectively towards shared goals.

During my nursing career, I've faced various instances of disrespect. One memory stands out when someone outrightly states, "I do not have to respect you." This provoked intense anger in me, almost leading to an altercation before another nurse intervened and stopped me. I also remember a charge nurse shouting, "Shut Up" at me. Such forms of disrespect should not be tolerated without addressing them with the supervisor. It's crucial to recognize when you're unable to address it yourself and escalate the issue to a supervisor or manager. Allowing oneself to be disrespected without addressing the problem only perpetuates the behavior. By taking proactive steps to address disrespect, we can effectively nip it in the bud and foster a culture of mutual respect within the workplace.

Why Improve Your Problem-solving skills?

In nursing, it's imperative to continually enhance problem-solving skills, as challenges frequently arise in patient care settings. Being proactive in identifying these challenges is key; once recognized, employing problem-solving abilities becomes essential in devising effective solutions. Collaboration with fellow team members can offer diverse perspectives and innovative ideas, particularly in patient care scenarios. Challenges are inherent to the nursing profession, necessitating the application of evidence-based practices learned in education to resolve them. Every nurse possesses inherent problem-solving abilities, often guided by intuition, and acquired knowledge. Sharing ideas and collaborating with colleagues enriches problem-solving approaches, leading to comprehensive solutions beneficial to patient care.

While some problems may require time and deliberation to solve, being methodical and strategic in approach facilitates successful resolution. Embracing problem-solving as an integral part of nursing not only enhances individual proficiency but also contributes to effective teamwork and optimal patients.

As a nurse, you will encounter numerous challenges. The best approach is to identify the issue, assess the potential solutions, determine the timeframe for resolution, and consider if additional resources are needed. Each time you successfully resolve a problem, it enhances your problem-solving skills, as similar issues are likely to arise again. While problem-solving isn't always straightforward and you may not always find a solution, having a supportive team can provide valuable guidance based on their past experiences.

For instance, I once faced a scheduling issue in dialysis where a patient urgently needed an extra treatment, but the schedule was full. By exploring options such as checking for cancellations, arranging a swap with another patient, or adjusting the schedule, you can effectively address patients' needs and enhance your problem-solving abilities through evidence-based practice. Outcomes.

Why Demonstrate Professionalism As A Team Member

It is imperative to uphold professionalism across all facets of your work, encompassing the maintenance of integrity, adherence to nursing ethics, and a sense of accountability. As a professional, it is vital to present yourself as the ideal candidate for the job, instilling confidence in your capabilities and reliability as a registered nurse or licensed practical nurse. This is also true for anyone working in the medical field. Your demeanor and communication with patients play a crucial role in their perception of care. When addressing patients, it is essential to do so in a professional manner, introducing yourself, explaining your purpose, the planned course of action, and the expected outcome. Maintaining professionalism not only influences how you are perceived by others but also sets a standard for your team members. It showcases your qualities, effectiveness in teamwork, communication skills, and commitment to improving patient care and fostering a positive work environment. As a professional nurse, you embody the essence of nursing and serve as a role model for others in the field.

Being professionals in the nursing field, our attire holds significant importance. I believe that our uniforms should be meticulously ironed and pressed, ensuring a neat and tidy appearance. Moreover, comfort is paramount, especially considering the physical demands of our job, which often involve bending and squatting. It's crucial to select attire that facilitates movement while maintaining professionalism. This aspect becomes even more pertinent when considering that we care for individuals of all genders.

Therefore, uniforms should not be overly tight, as they should reflect our dedication to professionalism without compromising comfort. In today's nursing landscape, there's a prevalent trend of tight-fitting scrubs, but I prefer a more traditional approach. My personal preference leans towards slightly loose attire, as it helps avoid attracting undue attention and fosters a sense of professionalism.

Additionally, a well-maintained uniform speaks volumes about one's commitment to their role. While some may argue that creases are unnecessary, I find that ensuring our attire is crisp and presentable enhances our overall professional image. Our choice of attire should aim to minimize distractions and maintain focus on providing optimal care to our patients.

How Do You Ensure Accountability as A Team Member?

Take ownership of your responsibilities and commitments within the team. Deliver high-quality work, meet deadlines, and fulfill your role to the best of your abilities. Hold yourself accountable for your actions and decisions and be proactive in addressing any issues or obstacles that may arise. As a team member it is important that you are accountable for your action. Whether the outcome are good or bad. Be accountable for your workload. When given assignments project try to complete them on time.

It is beneficial to outline your needs for a project and determine the timeline for completion upon receiving an appointment. I have always treated my assignments like a race against time, striving to finish them promptly and diligently. Accountability is essential in ensuring timely completion, both individually and as a team member.

Collaborating with others on assignments or projects requires fulfilling your responsibilities promptly, especially when different team members handle various sections. In nursing school, I experienced successful online project collaboration by dividing tasks, appointing a leader, and completing our respective parts. This approach facilitated easy assembly of the final project from everyone's contributions.

CHAPTER V

SHOWING EMPATHY & COMPASSION AS A NURSE

INTRODUCTION

Empathy, the profound ability to share the feelings of another, is a cornerstone of human connection and understanding. The empath, often referred to as the sensitive soul or the compassionate listener, possesses a remarkable capacity to step into the shoes of others, experiencing their joys and sorrows as if they were their own. In a world often fraught with misunderstandings and divisions, empathy offers solace, support, and understanding to those in need. Whether it's consoling a friend in distress, lending a listening ear to a stranger's woes, or championing causes for social justice and equality. Yet, despite these challenges, the empath's gift remains a precious asset in fostering deeper connections, promoting understanding, and cultivating a more empathetic world.

Why Is It Important To Have Empathy and Compassion?

In the healthcare profession, cultivating empathy and compassion towards both patients and colleagues is paramount. Understanding and acknowledging the emotions of patients can often be challenging, yet it is an essential aspect of providing holistic care. As professionals, it is crucial to recognize and validate the feelings of patients, offering them the support they need during challenging times.

Demonstrating empathy involves actively listening to patients as they express their concerns, asking open-ended questions to facilitate deeper understanding, and refraining from passing judgment. Non-verbal cues such as body language and facial expressions can also provide valuable insights into a patient's emotional state, allowing healthcare providers to respond appropriately.

By empathizing with patients' experiences and actively engaging in their interests and concerns, healthcare professionals can foster a sense of trust and compassion. Moreover, incorporating empathy into decision-making processes can help prioritize the well-being of both individuals and the broader community. By consistently demonstrating empathy and compassion, healthcare providers can create a supportive environment that promotes healing and patient-centered care.

Many times, patients may simply need to vent and share personal issues about their families or friends. At times, you may feel that this information isn't directly relevant or wonder why they're sharing it with you. However, as a nurse, it's crucial to demonstrate empathy and compassion by listening attentively, as these concerns are significant to the patients and may be causing them distress. Even if you have other tasks to attend to, taking the time to listen can make a meaningful difference to the patient. It's not always necessary to offer your opinion or thoughts; sometimes, patients just need someone to listen, which can alleviate their stress and make them feel understood. By showing empathy, you convey that their concerns matter to you as well, rather than dismissing their feelings. I've often found that simply listening to patients has been incredibly beneficial for them and has strengthened our nurse-patient relationship.

How Do Active Listening Show Compassion and Empathy?

Active listening for your patients shows them that you understand their fears, concerns, and emotions. This can be achieved through techniques such as maintaining eye contact, nodding to indicate understanding, and using validation methods to acknowledge their feelings. By actively listening, patients recognize that their nurse is attentive and responsive to their needs, fostering trust and rapport in the nurse-patient relationship.

This approach also applies to interactions with colleagues and interdisciplinary team members. By demonstrating genuine concern and attentiveness during discussions about patient care or treatment plans, nurses convey respect and validation for their teammates' perspectives. This collaborative approach promotes effective communication and enhances teamwork within the healthcare setting.

Sometimes letting the patient know that you understand how the situation is difficult for them ensures them that you know their emotions are valid sometimes just a simple compassionate touch can provide comfort for the patient reassuring them during a moment of distress or vulnerability holding their hand or gentle pat on the shoulder provides comfort sometimes a hug may even be appropriate.

How To Show Empathy and Compassion in Diverse Cultures

Understanding a patient's culture is paramount in demonstrating compassion. This emphasizes the significance of comprehending cultural nuances and practices, highlighting the importance of valuing diversity in patient care. Each patient, hailing from diverse backgrounds, adheres to unique routines and preferences. Displaying empathy towards their concerns, especially when they differ from familiar practices, is essential.

Similarly, this principle applies to interactions with colleagues of varying cultural backgrounds. Avoiding judgment and negative remarks regarding differences in behavior or dietary choices fosters a supportive and inclusive work environment. Acknowledging that diverse cultures have distinct rituals and routines underscores the essence of compassion in patient care. This underscores the need to recognize cultural differences, especially when patients struggle to articulate their needs in English. Employing gestures or repeating information demonstrates a commitment to understanding and accommodating their cultural perspectives, enhancing the quality of care provided.

When working with patients from diverse lifestyles, it's essential to acknowledge and respect their cultural beliefs, even if they differ from our own values and morals. Some cultures, particularly those with specific gender identities, may require sensitive handling to ensure they receive quality care and feel respected. While you might personally disagree with certain aspects of a patient's lifestyle, such as their preferred names or pronouns, as a nurse, it's vital to prioritize the patient's needs and preferences. Regardless of whether these lifestyle norms align with your beliefs, showing empathy and compassion towards all patients, regardless of their lifestyle background, is fundamental to providing equitable care. Every patient deserves to be treated with respect and receive the same level of care, regardless of differences or personal beliefs.

It's crucial to exhibit empathy and compassion towards your team members. Working closely with them exposes you to their various routines, preferences in activities, food choices, and communication styles. Therefore, showing understanding for their concerns, being patient with their difficulty in expressing themselves, and respecting their privacy when they're hesitant to discuss personal matters are essential aspects of fostering a supportive work environment. Additionally, regardless of whether you approve of their lifestyles, it's important to treat all coworkers with equal respect and empathy, acknowledging and empathizing with the challenges and experiences they face in their lives.

How Can Effective Documentation Show Empathy and Compassion?

Detailed documentation of patient's unique needs and preferences can help the providers in their approach to care displayed by acknowledging and respecting their patient space. An effective documentation is communication between the health care providers allowing them to maintain a consistency of the patient's needs and concerns.

Also, documentation can help the patient participate actively in discussions, treatment plans, and care instructions. It empowers patients to actively participate in their healthcare journey. When patients can review and understand their medical records, they feel more involved in decision-making processes, fostering a sense of agency and control.

Documentation serves as a means of communication and collaboration among healthcare team members. Clear and concise records facilitate effective information sharing, enabling providers to coordinate care seamlessly. This collaborative approach ensures that all team members are aligned in their understanding of the patient's needs, promoting a consistent and empathetic approach to care delivery.

Documenting the contributions and achievements of team members acknowledges their efforts and expertise. Recognizing their valuable contributions fosters a sense of appreciation and validation, promoting a supportive and empathetic work environment. Documenting feedback, mentorship sessions, or opportunities for professional development demonstrates a commitment to the growth and success of team members.

By having constructive feedback and guidance, documentation supports the ongoing learning of your development as a team member. This investment in your professional growth reflects empathy by showing a genuine interest in your well-being and career advancement. Documenting constructive feedback or praise for your work shows empathy by acknowledging your strengths, areas for improvement, and professional growth. Clear and respectful feedback demonstrates that the mentor values your development and well-being.

CHAPTER VI

HOW TO HAVE FLEXIBILITY AS A NURSING

INTRODUCTION

Central to this adaptability is the concept of flexibility in nursing practice. Flexibility in nursing encompasses a multifaceted approach, ranging from scheduling arrangements to clinical skills and interdisciplinary collaboration. It empowers nurses to navigate complex scenarios with agility, ensuring optimal patient care while fostering professional growth and resilience within the nursing workforce. In this era of rapid technological advancements, shifting demographics, and emerging healthcare challenges, the demand for flexible nursing practices has never been more pronounced. Nurses are expected to respond swiftly to fluctuations in patient acuity, embrace innovative technologies, from flexible scheduling models that promote work-life balance to adaptable clinical skills that accommodate diverse patient needs, flexibility in nursing serves as a catalyst for innovation, efficiency, and compassionate care.

Why is Adaptability Important In Nursing?

In the fast-paced landscape of today's medical field, the ability to adapt to change is paramount. Each year brings forth numerous alterations, making it imperative to remain flexible to navigate the evolving landscape effectively. This adaptability is particularly crucial when interacting with patients, managing workloads, and responding to managerial requirements.

Flexibility is essential, as schedules may need adjustment due to unforeseen circumstances or changes in staffing. Shift rotations are subject to modification, necessitating a mindset capable of accommodating such shifts. Furthermore, nurses must be prepared to seamlessly transition to different units or roles within the hospital setting as staffing needs fluctuate.

Adaptability extends beyond individual responsibilities to encompass interactions with managers and patients alike. Managers may need to adjust their teaching styles based on the staff's needs, while patient education may require tailoring to suit diverse cultural backgrounds. Adaptability plays a pivotal role in ensuring the smooth progression of patient care and fostering positive outcomes.

During my time as a new nurse on the units, I often experienced being floated to different units, such as transitioning from working on the Med-Surg unit to being assigned to the cardiac unit one night or Pediatrics on another night. As a nurse, it's crucial to adapt to these changes in patient care situations, given the constant fluctuations.

I had to learn to be flexible when facing short-staffed situations, adjusting to changes in patient loads or assignments that could occur frequently. For instance, there was an occasion when there was another outpatient facility that was understaffed and needed a charge nurse, I was sent by my director to take charge there for a month. The workflow and routines were different from what I was accustomed to, necessitating my adaptation to their methods despite the shared policies within the company. These instances highlight the importance of nurses being prepared to adapt to different units or critical situations that may arise unexpectedly in whether an outpatient or hospital setting, where emergencies or staffing shifts can occur, requiring flexibility and adaptability from all team members.

What Is The Significance Of Having Emotional Resilience?

Emotional resilience is indispensable in nursing, given the profession's emotionally taxing nature. Nurses confront a myriad of emotions daily, ranging from joy to grief, frustration, and compassion fatigue. Equipping nurses with emotional resilience is essential as it enables them to cope with the stressors inherent in their roles and mitigates the risk of burnout, safeguarding their well-being.

In emergencies, emotionally resilient nurses remain composed, effectively managing pressure and delivering compassionate care to patients. Such resilience is vital because a stressed or emotionally drained nurse cannot effectively serve patients or collaborate with their team.

Additionally, emotional resilience fosters strong interpersonal relationships with patients, families, and colleagues, promoting trust and collaboration in the work environment. By mastering emotional management, you will be able to enhance self-awareness, develop coping mechanisms, and cultivate resilience that extends beyond the workplace.

Furthermore, emotional resilience is crucial in navigating interactions with your team members and managers, ensuring continued effectiveness and job satisfaction despite challenges or conflicts. Overall, emotional resilience is fundamental to your nursing practice, enabling you to fulfill your duties effectively while maintaining personal well-being.

Maintaining emotional stability is crucial when working as a nurse, given the frequent encounters with emotionally challenging situations during your workday. How you manage these crises significantly impacts your effectiveness in nursing practice. There will be instances when patients display aggression or hostility, and your emotional response plays a pivotal role in handling such situations effectively. Failure to maintain emotional balance can lead to job dissatisfaction, feelings of overwhelm, and even thoughts of quitting.

Similarly, if you experience ongoing stress or conflict with teammates, it's important to address these issues with the management or seek support from mental health departments available in many workplaces. Keeping these discussions confidential, these resources can help prevent emotional distress, burnout, or health issues that may arise from prolonged emotional strain. Prioritizing your emotional resilience and seeking assistance when needed is essential for maintaining well-being and fulfilling your duties effectively in the nursing profession.

What Makes Multitasking Important In Nursing?

As nurses sometimes you have to be able to juggle multiple tasks at the same time in order to care for your patients I mean you'd have to do medication administration do vital signs attend to the patient needs treatments communicate with doctors other health professionals that might be there and sometimes this means you have to multitask in order to keep up the task of the day. Learning to multitask is so important because sometimes you have to be able to do an assessment really quick or assess the needs of multiple patients at one time because you're being called between the two patients and interventions are needed and this will help not delay the interventions that the patients made me multitasking can also help the nurse manage their time allowing them to allocate other resources this is essential for healthcare settings where nurses are responsible for caring for multiple patients. Sometime multitasking you find yourself communicating with the patients the patients' families other care professionals while you're doing your clinical task, so this also means you need to have effective communication to coordinate all this care that is needed.

 Learning how to multitask effectively is crucial for nurses as it enables them to evenly distribute their workload throughout shifts. However, effective multitasking requires a well-established system to manage tasks while remaining responsive to changes in patient conditions. This approach helps prevent complications and reduces the risk of medical errors. It's important to note that not everyone excels at multitasking, and some individuals may prefer focusing on one task at a time, which is also valid. Nonetheless, mastering multitasking skills can significantly enhance productivity and efficiency during the workday for nurses.

There may come a time when you are compelled to multitask, as I experienced while working on a surgical floor. I had two patients in the room, each needing their dressings changed. The situation became challenging when both doctors entered the room simultaneously, each requesting supplies and attention for their patient's dressing changes. This scenario highlights instances where you have no choice but to multitask, even if you prefer not to.

Why Is It Important For Nurses To Embrace Shift Work In Their Profession?

When planning for a nursing job, typically, you choose the shifts and hours you prefer to work. However, there are times when staffing shortages occur due to illness or other reasons, leading to an inadequate patient-to-nurse ratio. During such times, you must be willing to work different shifts, including days, nights, evenings, and weekends, and sometimes put in overtime to ensure the team functions effectively and delivers quality patient care. Being flexible with weekends and holidays is also important; coworkers may need time off, and being willing to switch shifts or alternate holidays helps maintain a harmonious work environment and supports the needs of the team.

As a charge nurse and a manager, rotating holidays among staff members is essential to prevent any individual from consistently working the same holiday every year, which could cause scheduling conflicts and impact morale. Flexibility in shift work and holiday scheduling is crucial for the smooth operation of healthcare teams. This also demonstrates your commitment to the team.

As a charge nurse, I ordered a large calendar for the bulletin board at the organization. This allowed us to track staff vacations and days off, preventing conflicts where everyone requested the same time off. Additionally, we required written vacation requests kept in a book to monitor holiday and vacation patterns. This organizational system ensured fairness and minimized conflicts over scheduling. Flexibility with shift times is crucial to maintain this organized approach.

CHAPTER VII

HOW CONTINUING EDUCATION HELP NURSES

INTRODUCTION

Continuing education is a cornerstone of excellence in nursing practice, ensuring that healthcare professionals remain at the forefront of advancements in patient care, technology, and evidence-based practices. In today's rapidly evolving healthcare landscape, where new treatments, procedures, and technologies emerge with increasing frequency, the commitment to lifelong learning is paramount for nurses to deliver high-quality care and uphold the highest standards of professionalism.

The nursing profession is multifaceted, encompassing a diverse range of specialties and practice settings, each with its unique challenges and opportunities. From acute care settings to community health, from pediatric to geriatric care, nurses play a critical role in promoting health, preventing illness, and caring for individuals across the lifespan. As the demands on the healthcare system evolve and patient needs become more complex, nurses must continually expand their knowledge, refine their skills, and adapt to new roles and responsibilities. Continuing education in nursing serves as a catalyst for professional growth, empowering nurses to stay abreast of current trends, best practices, and regulatory requirements.

What Are The Reasons For Attending Workshops and Conferences In Nursing?

Attending workshops and conferences holds myriad benefits for nurses, making them invaluable opportunities for professional development and personal growth. One primary reason is the imperative for continued education, given the rapid advancements across nursing technologies, treatments, and practices. These events afford nurses the chance to stay abreast of the latest developments and evidence-based practices shaping the nursing profession today.

Workshops and conferences serve as vital platforms for networking, allowing nurses to connect with peers, experts, and leaders from diverse backgrounds and specialties. This networking opportunity not only fosters collaboration but also opens doors for career advancement.

Conferences offer avenues for enhancing skills, competencies, and knowledge through hands-on training, skill-building workshops, and informative seminars. Exposure to innovative ideas, innovations, and improvements in patient care further enriches the learning experience, empowering nurses to adapt to evolving healthcare environments.

Attending these webinars, conferences, and workshops is crucial for gaining deeper insights into facility operations. Despite occasionally being away from the unit, you will find immense value in attending these events. They not only expand your understanding of patient care interventions but also allow you to acquire additional titles and roles, aside from being a nurse, due to the knowledge gained from these sessions.

Participating in workshops is essential for your personal and professional growth, as it equips you with new skills and interventions vital for your development. Furthermore, these conferences provide you with opportunities to network with other nurses, sharing experiences and learning from different perspectives. Personally, you should make it a point to engage with nurses from different facilities during these conferences, broadening your understanding and making the experience enjoyable and enriching.

Additionally, many workshops and conferences offer educational credits, essential for maintaining nursing licensure and certifications.

Participation in such events underscores your commitment to the profession and long-term career growth. Attending complementary healthcare facilities workshops helps by providing you with crucial updates on hospital practices and procedures. These sessions serve as refresher courses, ensuring you remain well-equipped to deliver high-quality patient care and collaborate effectively within interdisciplinary teams. Attending workshops and conferences is not just about learning the latest practices in nursing; it's about investing in one's professional and personal growth, enriching both the individual nurse and the broader healthcare community.

During my time working in the hospital, attending end services was mandatory, leaving us with no choice but to participate. This turned out to be a valuable learning experience, as it involved vendors coming in to educate us about their supplies and new products beneficial for patient care. Similarly, when I transitioned to an outpatient facility in dialysis, the manager recognized my interest in learning more about the facility and started taking me to various conferences with her. These experiences exposed me to a wealth of knowledge and opportunities for professional development.

How Does Reading Nursing Journals and Publications Benefit Your Nursing Profession?

Reading nursing journals and publications is highly beneficial for nurses as they provide the latest research findings and best practices for everyday clinical care. Staying updated with these publications enables nurses to incorporate the most effective and current interventions into their practice. Continuous learning is crucial in the nursing profession due to ongoing advancements in insights, technologies, treatments, and practices highlighted in these journals.

Engaging with nursing journals also helps contribute to your professional development by offering new insights, expanding knowledge bases, and improving critical thinking skills. Scholarly articles in these journals often emphasize critical thinking for you, aiding in quality improvement and keeping you informed about current trends and best practices. Additionally, subscribing to nursing magazines or journals on a regular basis helps you stay abreast of developments in your field, connect with expert peers, and contribute to quality improvement initiatives within your healthcare facilities.

Moreover, utilizing nursing journals as educational resources for patients is advantageous, as it empowers patients to take an active role in their health decisions based on evidence-based information. This practice not only aids in patient education but also supports you in acting as advocates for your patients and your profession.

During my early years as a nurse, I exclusively subscribed to the American Journal of Nursing. At that time, I wasn't aware of other nursing journals. Over time, my monthly subscription resulted in accumulating numerous magazines. Despite my initial interest in the subjects covered, such as patient care and treatment best practices, I eventually became too busy to read them all. As a result, the magazines started piling up in my house.

Nevertheless, subscribing to nursing journals is beneficial because they contain valuable information and insights about various aspects of nursing practice.

What Are The Benefits of Participating In Quality Improvement Programs In Nursing?

Getting involved in quality improvement initiatives can significantly enhance patient outcomes. These programs are designed to identify and implement best practices that lead to better patient care. By actively participating in quality improvement efforts, nurses contribute to the ongoing enhancement of care quality. Moreover, these initiatives play a crucial role in improving patient safety, addressing issues such as medical errors, adverse events, and infection control practices. By engaging in quality improvement activities, nurses can help reduce these events, ensuring that patients receive the highest quality of care and support they deserve.

Furthermore, quality improvement efforts focus on optimizing healthcare delivery workflows, making processes more efficient and effective. You can play a pivotal role in this aspect by identifying workflow inefficiencies, proposing improvements, and implementing changes to enhance patient care delivery. Participating in quality improvement programs also serves as a means of professional development for you, fostering leadership, teamwork, and problem-solving skills through active engagement in improvement projects.

Many healthcare organizations mandate staff participation in quality improvement to maintain accreditation and comply with regulatory standards. Your involvement in these programs ensures that organizations remain in good standing and continue to provide quality care. Quality improvement is a continuous process, involving ongoing monitoring, evaluation, and refinement of practices to achieve better outcomes.

By participating in quality improvement initiatives, you contribute to cultivating a culture of continuous improvement within your organizations, where learning and innovation are highly valued. Collaboration across disciplines is integral to these efforts, providing you with opportunities to work closely with other healthcare professionals, such as physicians, pharmacists, and administrators, to address various improvement needs within the facility.

While working as a charge nurse in an outpatient clinic, I was actively involved in quality improvement meetings as a committee member. My responsibilities included presenting monthly results and discussing strategies to enhance areas where our performance fell short of goals. Upon transitioning to a clinical manager role, I assumed greater responsibility by leading these meetings, documenting inputs from the multidisciplinary team, analyzing performance reports, and devising interventions to address shortcomings.

Upon returning to the hospital after my years in dialysis, I was assigned to another quality improvement team that operated with weekly meetings and assigned projects aimed at enhancing various aspects and metrics within the facility. Participating in these programs yielded several benefits, such as the opportunity to present innovative solutions during quality meetings, contributing to problem-solving efforts, and feeling a sense of pride in actively contributing to positive changes within the organization.

Is It Advisable to Become A Member Of A Professional Nursing Organization?

Joining a professional nursing organization offers numerous benefits for nurses, aiding in both career advancement and personal development. These organizations provide invaluable networking opportunities, connecting members with fellow nurses, healthcare professionals, educators, and industry leaders. Within these networks, you can find mentorship opportunities to further their professional growth. Additionally, membership grants access to a wealth of resources, including workshops, seminars, conferences, and the latest developments in nursing practice, enriching skills, and knowledge. Moreover, you can leverage their membership to advocate for the profession and patient care at local, national, or international levels, contributing to policymaking and legislation. Professional nursing organizations also enhance career visibility and demonstrate commitment to healthcare, opening doors to various career opportunities.

Furthermore, these organizations often engage in community outreach, addressing community needs and advocating for you as a nurse and patients alike. Overall, participation in nursing organizations offers diverse avenues for advocacy and professional development within your organization.

I initially joined the American Nurses Association during my student years and maintained my membership for a few years thereafter. Additionally, I became a member of the New Jersey Nurses Association. Although I couldn't attend their conferences, I stayed updated with their literature and subscribed to their emails, keeping me informed about the latest developments within the organization.

Both organizations actively participate in various advocacy efforts, including marches to Washington, where they advocate for nursing salaries, patient ratios, and overall equality within the profession. These organizations play a crucial role in advocating for the rights and interests of nurses across different platforms and initiatives. Nursing community.

HERE IS SOME NAMES OF NURSING ORGANIZATIONS:

1. **American Nurses Association (ANA)

2. **National League for Nursing (NLN)

3. **American Association of Critical-Care Nurses (AACN)

4. **Emergency Nurses Association (ENA)

5. **Association of Perioperative Registered Nurses (AORN)

6. **National Association of School Nurses (NASN)

7. **American Psychiatric Nurses Association (APNA)

8. **Association of Women's Health, Obstetric and Neonatal Nurses (AWHONN)

1. **National Black Nurses Association (NBNA)

2. **Black Nurses Rock (BNR)

3. **Black Nurses Association of Greater Washington, D.C. Area (BNA of GWDC)

4. **National Association of Hispanic Nurses (NAHN)

5. **National Coalition of Ethnic Minority Nurse Associations (NCEMNA)

6. American Association of Colleges of Nursing (AACN)

CHAPTER VIII

ETHICAL AND LEGAL CONSIDERATIONS IN NURSING

INTRODUCTION

In the dynamic and challenging field of nursing, nurses are confronted with numerous ethical and legal dilemmas daily. The decisions nurses make not only impact patient care but also have implications for their professional standing and the healthcare system. Understanding and navigating these ethical and legal considerations are paramount to delivering safe, effective, and compassionate care.

Ethical considerations in nursing encompass a range of principles. These principles, including beneficence, nonmaleficence, autonomy, and justice, provide a framework for nurses to uphold the highest standards of ethical conduct in their practice. Ethical conduct may arise when balancing the rights of patients, respecting confidentiality, and adhering to professional boundaries.

Legal considerations in nursing pertain to the laws, regulations, and standards that govern the profession. Nurses must be well-versed in their legal responsibilities, such as maintaining patient confidentiality, obtaining informed consent, and documenting care accurately. Failure to adhere to legal requirements can result in disciplinary action, legal consequences, and jeopardize patient safety.

Why Is It Important to Know About Ethical and legal Considerations in Nursing?

Knowing about ethical and legal considerations in nursing is crucial for several reasons:

As the nurse you are responsible for the patient's safety and well-being. When you decide to care for the patient, you must make sure it's in the patient's best interest. You want the patient to have trust in your judgement. You must adhere to regulations and standards of patient care. This will help you avoid disciplinary actions and litigations.

As a new nurse you must locate these rules and regulations in your facility or unit that gives you information on the legal and ethical principles of patient care. Every facility that I have worked t conducts monthly rounds just to make sure that the units have patient rights and regulations hanging on the wall for all employees to see.

What Are Ethical Principles in Nursing Practice?

Ethical principles in nursing practice are fundamental guidelines that help nurses make ethical decisions and navigate complex moral dilemmas in patient care. You are expected to respect the patient's rights to make their own decision about the treatments they are receiving. This is the principle of autonomy. You are expected to strive for the patient's well-being by promoting improved patient outcomes. You should make sure the patient is protected under your care by minimizing negative consequences. All patients should be treated fairly by you no matter what their culture or beliefs are. You should give patients information honestly about their treatments. Most of all maintain your integrity and adhere to nursing standards.

When I was caring for patients, the moment I walked in the room, I informed them about what my intents were. I answered any questions they asked and told them the truth based on my scope of practice. If I didn't know something, I let them know I would find out and come back to them with the information. In information out of my scope of practice, I informed them to save it for their doctor.

What Are The Legal Obligations and Responsibilities In The Nursing Practice?

While working as a nurse, you are legally responsible for maintaining a current nursing license in the state where you practice. Specialty areas in nursing may require certification. Before you do any treatment or intervention with the patient or any procedure, you should get informed consent from the patient. As the nurse, you should advocate making this a practice for every patient, no matter what department comes in to do a procedure, X-ray, or EKG. The nurse is responsible for ensuring the patient consented to treatments. The Joint Commission advocates for the patients to make sure that the patient, understand fully what their treatment options are, the risks or the benefits of receiving these interventions. You are responsible for all legal documentation, such as assessment, medication, intervention, and any medical records that pertain to the patient.

As a nurse involved in risk management, you are tasked with identifying potential risks for patients, such as falls, infections, medication errors, and other adverse events. It is crucial to report all adverse events promptly. In your role as an organizing nurse, you hold responsibility for overseeing all aspects of patient care during their stay, regardless of the treatments or interventions they require. This means that as a nurse, everything concerning the patient's well-being falls under your license while they are under your care.

Why Is Patient Confidentiality and Privacy Important in Nursing?

As a nurse responsible for a patient's care, maintaining confidentiality and respecting their privacy is important. Discussing patient information, medical records, or treatment details in public areas such as elevators or hallways where others might overhear violates patient confidentiality and privacy rights. When admitting patients to the hospital, refrain from sharing their information with outside parties unless authorized by the patient or their legal representative.

Under HIPAA laws, nurses must obtain written consent or permission from patients before disclosing any medical records to individuals, including family members. Even if a patient shares personal details during conversations, unless it directly impacts their medical care or interventions, this information remains confidential between the nurse and the patient.

Building trust and rapport with patients is essential for effective care. Patients who trust their nurses are more likely to disclose valuable information and collaborate on their treatment plans. However, it's crucial to maintain professionalism by adhering to HIPAA regulations and respecting patients' rights to privacy.

CHAPTER IX

NAVIGATING THE PATH OF NURSING ENTREPPRENEUSHIP

INTRODUCTION

As healthcare evolves and demands innovative solutions, the role of nurses extends beyond traditional clinical settings. Nursing entrepreneurship has emerged as a dynamic avenue for nurses to leverage their expertise, creativity, and passion for patient care while exploring entrepreneurial opportunities.

Nursing entrepreneurship encompasses a wide range of activities, including starting and managing healthcare businesses, developing innovative products or services, consulting, coaching, and advocating for healthcare reforms. Nurses in entrepreneurial roles leverage their clinical knowledge, leadership skills, and business acumen to address healthcare challenges, improve patient outcomes, and drive positive change within the industry.

What Is The Challenges of Nursing Entrepreneurship?

Embarking on the path of nursing entrepreneurship comes with its unique set of challenges and opportunities. You may encounter hurdles such as navigating regulatory requirements, securing funding, managing financial risks, building a client base, and balancing clinical expertise with business acumen. However, if you decide to get into nursing entrepreneurship, it offers opportunities for autonomy, creativity, professional growth, and the ability to make a meaningful impact on healthcare delivery and patient experiences. You will become your own boss and make your own rules, that others must abide by. You know longer work by a set time frame. Your hours can be flexible.

What Does It Take To Be A Successful Entrepreneur In Nursing?

To establish a thriving nursing business, meticulous planning and strategic execution are imperative. First, you must possess the requisite skills and expertise in your chosen area of business. Understanding your target clients and defining the specific areas of focus within your expertise is crucial. Before venturing into entrepreneurship, drafting a comprehensive business plan is essential. This plan should encompass your vision, goals, marketing strategies, financial projections, and operational processes.

Building a network and fostering collaborations within the industry are equally important. Engaging with peers and industry stakeholders not only provides insights into industry trends but also helps in leveraging partnerships, enhancing visibility, and establishing credibility. Keeping abreast of emerging trends and advancements in marketing strategies relevant to your business is vital.

Developing a strong brand identity and effectively promoting your services or products is key to attracting clients. Clearly communicating your offerings to clients is essential for building a loyal customer base. Maintaining sound financial management practices, including tracking revenue and managing expenses, is fundamental to the success of your business.

Many nurses are opening nursing agencies for home care. You must adhere to legal and ethical standards is non-negotiable. Ensuring compliance with regulations, securing necessary licenses, and addressing liabilities and insurance are critical aspects of running a nursing business ethically and legally. Upholding high standards of professionalism and ethical conduct not only safeguards your business but also builds trust and credibility with clients and stakeholders. It is good to know there are options to working at the bedside in nursing.

CHAPTER X

THE BUSINESS THAT ALMOST WAS!

My goal was to open a home care agency when I retire. It did not become known due to financial reasons. Here is my Story:

Why did I want to start a business?

One of my family members who is an LPN, brought the suggestion to me. Every time she saw me, she was bringing it up. During the time when I was working in dialysis, one of my dialysis patients asked me, "Avalon, when are you going to retire? What are you going to do?" I said, "Well, a family member wants to start a home health agency." He said, "Oh, my wife, she has her own home health agency. She could help you with all of that if you're interested. I could set you all up for dinner and she'll tell you what you need to do." He called his wife, he set us up for dinner, and she gave us all the information on what it would take to start the business. I took notes on everything that we would need to do to start this home health agency. Once we found out what was needed to start, we just took the information and started the process.

What skills did I have to start a business and make it successful?

First, you really need to have some background knowledge of the health care system. If you're going to do home health agency, like we were going to do, you need some nursing background, because without that I don't think you would be able to meet the client's needs. Having a nursing background is important. You must be able to ensure that you make the patients feel you're confident in what you're doing. You must show you or your agency can meet their needs. And they need to know you are the professional person who will take care of them. Their family must feel comfortable enough that you're a professional caregiver and they don't have to worry about their family members. The patient must feel confident that you know what you are doing. These are the type of things you need to be successful.

What are five tips you can give an aspiring nurse entrepreneur that will help them monetize their business online?

I believe you should have at least some connections with others who have started the type of business that you are looking to get into. Become familiar with what they're doing so that they can help you have at least an outline or plan for your business. Explore the internet, look for information, do some research, and find out information on the type of business you want to start. Once you do your research, find out how you can move forward with what you're planning to do. Attend some seminars. There are a lot of seminars out there regarding home health care. Attend some of them, take notes, and put things in motion. Those are things that can help monetize a person's business.

What challenges have you had to overcome in your business?

My biggest challenge was financial. We got the business started, and we had everything in place. We were licensed. We went through the city inspection without a problem. Then COVID hit. Once COVID hit, we decided that because COVID was so unknown at the time, we weren't comfortable going into clients' houses. So, we held off for an entire year. Then next year we're going to start back up. Before we could resume the business, we had to renew everything because everything had expired, I noticed that money was starting to be missing out of the business account. Once that happened, it turned me off from wanting to continue the business, and I just backed out. It was a financial challenge for me.

Who is your ideal client? And why do you need an ideal client?

For me, the ideal client is the one that has exceptionally good family support. Because if they have a good supportive family, then you know that the family is willing to be educated. They will be there to listen every time you educate the patient. They're interested in the patient's care. The patient is interested and wants to participate in what you educate them. You can teach the family how to be involved in the patient's care when you're not around. For me, that's the ideal patient, the one that has a supportive family. They care about what type of treatment the patient is getting. The patient cares about their treatment. That makes an ideal patient for me, that family support system.

When it comes to marketing for a business like yours, what advice can you give that will be helpful to aspiring nurse entrepreneurs? What was difficult for you in marketing?

Well, I didn't have the chance to get to the marketing part because of the financial issue and shutting it down. But for those that do get to that point, using social media and sending out press releases can help. Making flyers and campaign ads and hanging flyers up around various places. I know a lot of places may not want you to hang flyers up. But if they allow you to put those flyers up, have your family members and your friends pass the word around. They can also help pass out flyers or help do the campaigns with you. Go to your town newspapers. Some towns have resources when you open a business that they'll help you advertise your business. These are all the things. Any resources that you can use that's out there here, I would say use them all.

What motivated you to start such a business as yours?

Because I had at that time 38 years of nursing experience, and have worked in many areas of nursing, and was once certified as a Medical surgical nurse. I did many years of home care nursing I worked as a visiting nurse Per Diem. I work full-time in the hospital. I did a lot of private duty cases. I knew the clinical process, and how it worked. I just wasn't familiar with the business end, and that's the part I need to learn. I enjoyed doing home care. I enjoyed doing private duty. I felt like since I had knowledge in that field that this would be a good business to venture into. By the time I retire I will have extra income to look forward to. At least that was the plan.

What do you want to tell other women in nursing about starting a business?

Because of my experience in starting a business for me, I would say try to start your business alone. Only because having partners could cause issues like it did with me. Make sure your office is accessible near the bus line because not drive. So, your staff will be able to get there. You may be able to hire more people if the office is closer to a bus line. Do not enter a loan with a partner unless you know their financial stability. This way when it's time to repay the loan, you are not caught off guard with them saying, "I do not have it right now." It really took me for a loop that I ended up with the financial burden of this because of having a partner. I did not know the financial stability of the partner that I chose. If you do have a partner, make sure that you're keeping an eye on the business account because that's the mistake I made. I wasn't really watching it. Then when I decided to investigate it, that's when I started noticing that money was missing. Even though we were paying this loan together and we had this business together, the person was going into the business account, which they should have never touched.

Just make sure that you're keeping a watchful eye. Make sure the person you decide to have a partner with is as committed to the business as you are. Make sure you get an exceptionally good electronic system that keeps the patient's records. It's good to have, and they have so many systems out there to keep everything in order. We had bought a system that would do everything. My partner had worked as a medical assistant in the doctor's office and used the system. Just conduct exceptionally good backgrounds on your staff that you hire. That includes anybody that you're going to hire into your agency or company. Make sure that you're getting good background checks on them, and just try to get some sponsors to help you grow your business.

What types of tools are important when starting a business?

In the business that we were going to start, the tools that we needed, we had to be licensed. We needed a business plan. We had to make sure we had locked cabinets, we needed a good office in a suitable location, and we needed to be accredited. We had educational backgrounds and educational training tools for your staff, employee handbooks, policies and procedures, computers, we needed software, tax ID, and surety bonds. Different binders that pertained to the business. These are the types of tools that we need to start our business.

As a current business owner do you plan to expand your business?

Because of the experience I had, I do not want to pursue opening an agency anymore. Now, that's where my mind is. I have decided to become a full-time entrepreneur as an author. I will attend training classes to learn better marketing skills for my books. Increase advertisement on social media platforms. Visit libraries and daycares. Increase my appearances on podcast, radio, and broadcast. Atten speaking classes to reach my audiences.

Name at least five businesses a nurse can start today.

Nurses can start a home health agency, PICC line insertion agency, vascular access facilities, become midwives, and open a medical clinic.

Although I only name five areas where a nurse can start a business, there are so many other areas of nursing that are opening for those nurses who want to start their own business.

CONCLUSION

In conclusion, embarking on a journey in the nursing profession demands a multifaceted approach to preparation and continuous development. Researching the profession, conversing with fellow nurses, and understanding personal resilience to stress are fundamental steps in laying a solid foundation. Moreover, delineating long-term professional and personal goals provides a guiding light throughout one's career. Licensing, certificates, and degrees serve as benchmarks for competence and specialization, while transitioning from a student nurse to a professional requires adaptability and a commitment to lifelong learning. Creating a positive learning environment and promoting independence during mentorship foster growth and confidence among colleagues.

Critical thinking, prioritization of time-sensitive tasks, and appropriate delegation are crucial skills that streamline workflow and enhance patient care. Managing self-care ensures nurses remain physically and mentally fit to fulfill their duties effectively. Effective communication and mutual respect within the team bolster collaboration and foster a supportive work culture. Improving problem-solving skills and demonstrating professionalism underscore the dedication to delivering optimal patient outcomes. Empathy and compassion lie at the heart of nursing, exemplified through active listening, culturally sensitive care, and empathetic documentation. Adaptability, emotional resilience, and multitasking abilities are indispensable traits that enable nurses to navigate the dynamic healthcare landscape.

Engaging in workshops, reading nursing journals, and participating in quality improvement programs enriches knowledge and fosters professional growth. Finally, joining a professional nursing organization provides a platform for networking, advocacy, and continuous advancement within the field. Embracing these principles equips nurses to excel in their noble profession and make a meaningful impact on the lives of those they serve.

I hope that readers of this book will find valuable and relevant information that can contribute to their career growth in nursing. While this book covers several aspects of nursing, I aim to provide enough content for readers to consider nursing as a profession and understand the expectations associated with it. My goal is to offer insights that can help readers gain a better understanding of the nursing profession.

ABOUT THE AUTHOR

Author Avalon Soulette Brown is a #1 Best selling author from Newark, NJ. Avalon has over 42 years of experience in nursing. Eighteen years in GI/GU post-op surgical floor, twenty years of dialysis experience, where she held multiple titles. Charge nurse, Anemia Manager, Infection Control Nurse, Transplant Designee, Vascular Nurse, and a Clinical Manager. She's also worked in home care for three years. Avalon recently worked as an Infection Preventionist for 3 1/2 years. After working for over four-year decades Avalon retired and continues to write books.

In addition to being a nurse, Author Avalon Brown is #1 bestselling author from Newark, NJ. Avalon has written numerous children's books using her grandchildren as characters. These books will serve as her legacy for her family. Avalon has also written a spiritual poetry book, a bibliography of her father life as a bishop, and a memoir of her nursing career. Avalon is also a co-author of nine anthologies, including her own anthology, Nursing is Our Passion "We Can't Quit."

Avalon earned her LPN from Essex County Tech in Newark NJ. Her ASN is from Essex County College in Newark. Her BSN from Regis University in Colorado. She is a member of the American Nurses Association and Professional; Organization for Women of Excellence Recognized.

FB: Author Avalon S Brown

IG: @authoravalons

EM: authoravalonsbrown@yahoo.com

www.ingramcontent.com/pod-product-compliance
Lightning Source LLC
Chambersburg PA
CBHW070213230526
45471CB00002B/940